This Book
Belongs To:
_____

Don't Give Up

If you saw the
size of the
♡blessing♡
coming, you would
understand the
magnitude of
the battle
you are fighting.

❀ LITTLE ABOUT US ❀

Parents to be

Name ....   Name ....

Age ....   Age ....

Occupation ....   Occupation ....

Together since ....

How we met ....

....

....

INSERT PHOTO

We are doing IVF because...

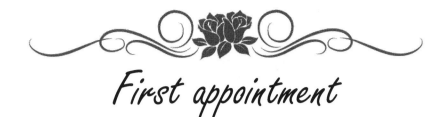

First appointment

CLINIC ....
NHS/PRIVATE ....
DOCTOR...
CONSULTATION APPOINTMENT: ....../....../......

How it went...

Treatment Plan

◯ LONG PROTOCOL

◯ SHORT PROTOCOL

Medication

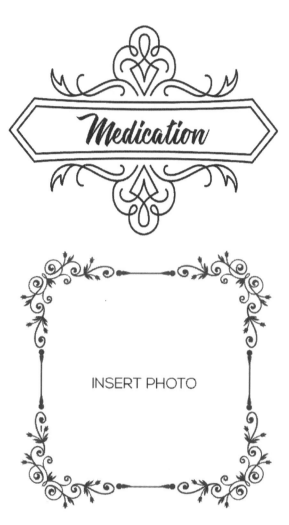

INSERT PHOTO

My cocktail of IVF meds is...

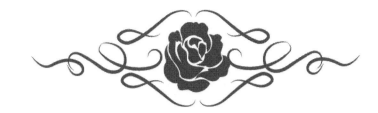

Gratitude & Feelings

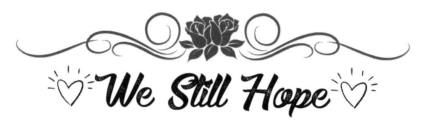

We Still Hope

And sometimes against all odds, against all logic, we still hope.

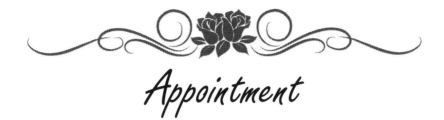

Appointment

CLINIC ....
NHS/PRIVATE ....
DOCTOR...
CONSULTATION APPOINTMENT: ....../....../.....

How it went...

Treatment Plan

◯   LONG PROTOCOL

◯   SHORT PROTOCOL

Medication

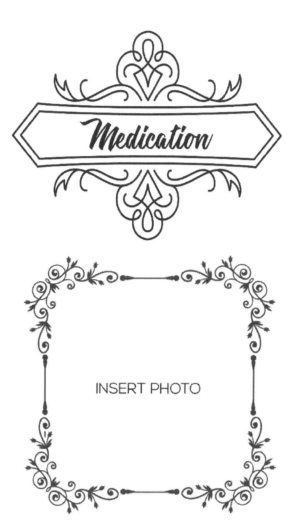

My cocktail of IVF meds is...

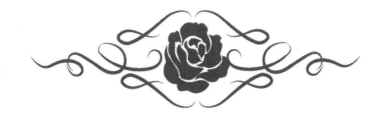

Gratitude & Feelings

....

....

....

....

....

....

....

....

....

....

....

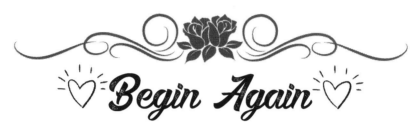

Begin Again

And you begin again and sometimes you lose, sometimes you win, but you begin again. Even though your heart is breaking, in time the sun will shine and you will begin again.

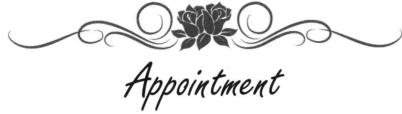

Appointment

CLINIC ....

NHS/PRIVATE ....

DOCTOR...

CONSULTATION APPOINTMENT: ...../...../.....

How it went...

Treatment Plan

○ LONG PROTOCOL

○ SHORT PROTOCOL

Medication

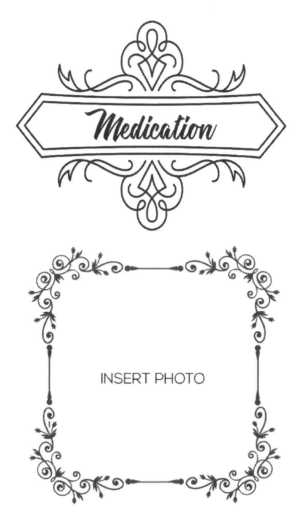

INSERT PHOTO

My cocktail of IVF meds is...

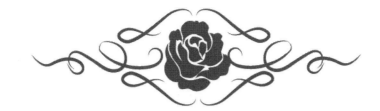

Gratitude & Feelings

....

....

....

....

....

....

....

....

....

....

....

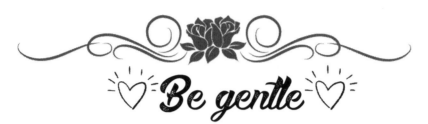

Be gentle with
yourself, you're
doing the best you
can.

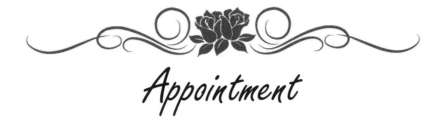

Appointment

CLINIC ....

NHS/PRIVATE ....

DOCTOR...

CONSULTATION APPOINTMENT: ....../....../......

> *How it went...*

Treatment Plan

○   LONG PROTOCOL

○   SHORT PROTOCOL

Medication

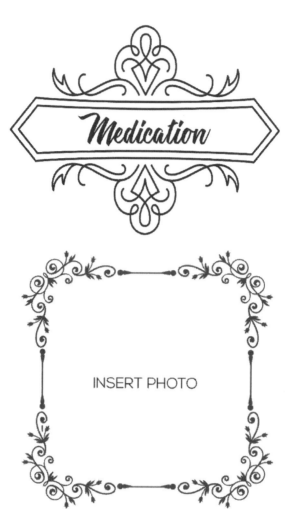

INSERT PHOTO

My cocktail of IVF meds is...

_____
_____
_____
_____
_____
_____

Gratitude & Feelings

....

....

....

....

....

....

....

....

....

....

....

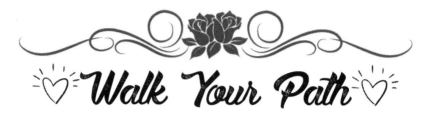

Walk Your Path

Don't expect
everyone to
understand your
journey
especially if they've
never had to walk your
path.

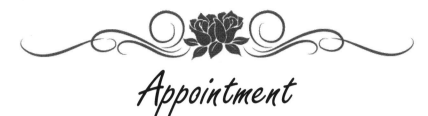

Appointment

CLINIC ....

NHS/PRIVATE ....

DOCTOR...

CONSULTATION APPOINTMENT: ....../....../......

How it went...

Treatment Plan

◯ LONG PROTOCOL

◯ SHORT PROTOCOL

Medication

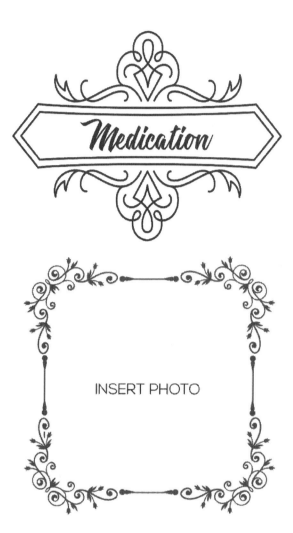

INSERT PHOTO

My cocktail of IVF meds is...

_____
_____
_____
_____
_____
_____

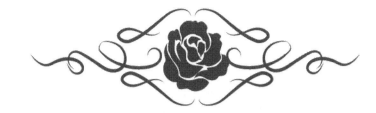

Gratitude & Feelings

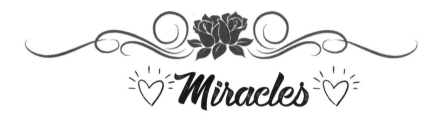

Even Miracles take a little time.

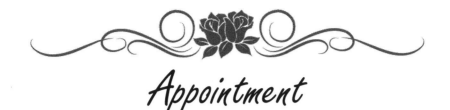

Appointment

CLINIC ....
NHS/PRIVATE ....
DOCTOR...
CONSULTATION APPOINTMENT: ....../....../......

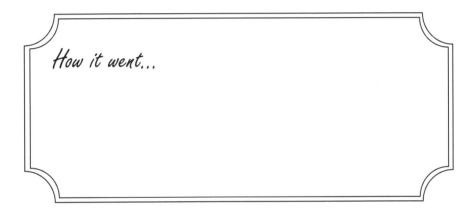

How it went...

Treatment Plan

◯   LONG PROTOCOL

◯   SHORT PROTOCOL

Medication

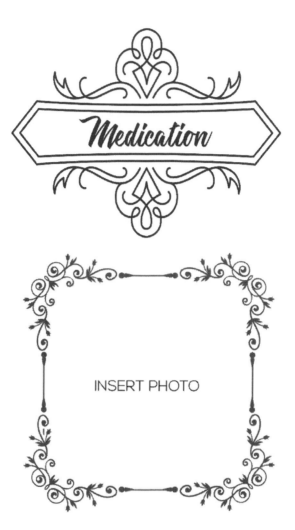

INSERT PHOTO

My cocktail of IVF meds is...

- -
- -
- -
- -
- -
- -

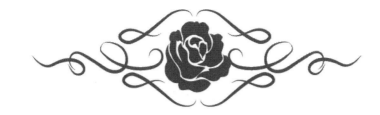

Gratitude & Feelings

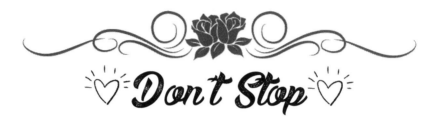

Don't Stop

If you can't stop
thinking about it,
don't stop
working for it.

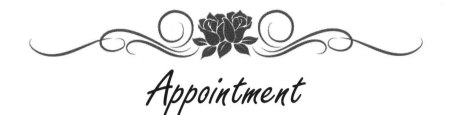

Appointment

CLINIC ....

NHS/PRIVATE ....

DOCTOR...

CONSULTATION APPOINTMENT: ....../....../......

How it went...

Treatment Plan

○ LONG PROTOCOL

○ SHORT PROTOCOL

Medication

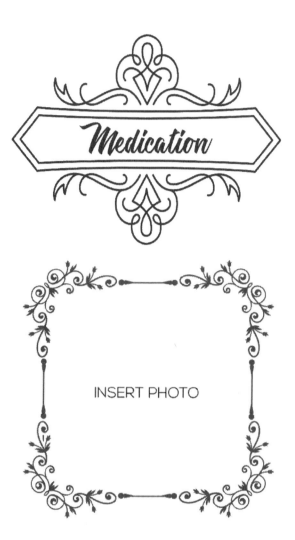

INSERT PHOTO

My cocktail of IVF meds is...

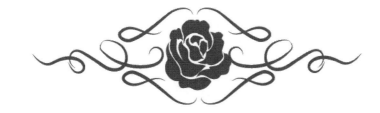

Gratitude & Feelings

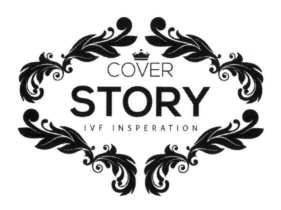

What separates those who seem to have all the 'luck' in the world versus those who just can't catch a break? What's the defining difference between these types of people? If you're an entrepreneur, you know the answer already. If you're just venturing into the unknown territory of *business* – this is a skill you will have to learn.

Yes, I'm calling **mindset** a learned skill. For some, it comes naturally. My husband John for example believes he was born a risk-taker, and always had an innate belief in himself. *Not everyone is John.* Some of us need a little help practicing believing in ourselves, day in and day out. John will tell you that he invests in his mindset every day – so while he may have been born with talent ...he's worked very hard fostering it, and continues to.

So when we were both hit with one of our **biggest marital challenges**, we were put to the test. Struggling with fertility issues is no walk in the park. It will challenge your way of thinking, make you question everything and search for answers that you may never find. I have seen it devastate women; I remember attending a non-profit event I hosted in honor of raising funds for female infertility *(and by the* *way I hate the word infertility because it seems so finite which is why I never used the term when describing my situation to others,* and witnessing the impact it had on the women who were still waiting, hopelessly – to have a family. I heard stories of women who felt that without the title

of **mother** – their life was *meaningless.*

What I do remember throughout my 3 + year journey to get to where I am today is believing that we would be parents someday. We didn't know when or even how – sort of like when building a business ...so much of it is a mystery, so much uncertainty. The only thing you have is your mindset, and your ability to cope with the shifting winds. The universe – or whatever you want to call it ...tested my faith time and time again, but I remember December 2016. I yelled out loud, *"You think you can break me? You can't break me!"*

And then not even a month later, I mustered myself up for another procedure – this time a surgery to slice me open to remove fibroids. I recovered quickly. I call this resiliency. I didn't have time to dwell. Keep going, no need to feel sorry

for **me**. I know how this story ends. I've written it down, it's on my vision boards – so don't worry about me. *I got this.* I'm not saying it was easy, and I'm not saying my armour protected me day in and day out. I had days ...dreadful days, but that voice – a soft whisper told me *"You'll be a mother someday."*

Throughout it all, my husband told me *"I'll love you no matter what. I didn't marry you so you could have my children."* This was incredibly freeing. I hope your soulmate believes the same for the two of you, because as women – we feel the pressures of society ...what our role should be in this world. But today, we are rewriting the rules.

So whether you want to be a mother or not, that should solely be your decision. And you shouldn't be ashamed by your choice or heart's desire one way or another.

Because I shared my personal journey through IVF with you (two failed rounds) and a fibroid removal surgery, I felt it only fair to let you in not only on my struggles in life but my triumphs.

The second round of IVF left us with *one embryo. Frozen in time*, we waited until it was our turn to try again.

And try again we did – because in life, you should never give up on the things you want. Whether it's parenthood, finding the love of your life, getting that degree, applying for your dream job, traveling the world, or building a business...

Do.Not.Give.Up.

The universe favors those who have persistent faith. And when you don't have faith? Borrow it. Because that's what I did...

At the end, we're 17 weeks pregnant and we're having a girl!

Written By *Nineveh Madsen*